CNA
Mentoring
Made
Easy

CNA
Mentoring
Made
Easy

Second Edition

Everything You Need to Run a
Successful Peer Mentoring Program

Karl Pillemer

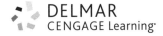

DELMAR
CENGAGE Learning·

Australia • Brazil • Japan • Korea • Mexico • Singapore • Spain • United Kingdom • United States

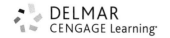
DELMAR
CENGAGE Learning·

CNA Mentoring Made Easy: Everything You Need to Run a Successful Peer Mentoring Program, Second Edition

Karl Pillemer

Vice President, Career and Computing: Dave Garza

Director of Learning Solutions: Matthew Kane

Senior Acquisitions Editor: Maureen Rosener

Managing Editor: Marah Bellegarde

Product Manager: Samantha L. Miller

Vice President, Career and Professional Marketing: Jennifer Ann Baker

Marketing Director: Wendy E. Mapstone

Senior Marketing Manager: Michele McTighe

Marketing Coordinator: Scott A. Chrysler

Senior Production Director: Wendy Troeger

Production Manager: Andrew Crouth

Content Project Manager: PreMediaGlobal

Senior Art Director: Jack Pendleton

Cover Image: courtesy of iStock.com

For product information and technology assistance, contact us at **Cengage Learning Customer & Sales Support, 1-800-354-9706**

For permission to use material from this text or product, submit all requests online at **www.cengage.com/permissions**. Further permissions questions can be e-mailed to **permissionrequest@cengage.com**.

Library of Congress Control Number: 2011943875

ISBN-13: 978-1-133-27780-4

ISBN-10: 1-133-27780-2

Delmar
5 Maxwell Drive
Clifton Park, NY 12065-2919
USA

Cengage Learning is a leading provider of customized learning solutions with office locations around the globe, including Singapore, the United Kingdom, Australia, Mexico, Brazil, and Japan. Locate your local office at: **international.cengage.com/region**

Cengage Learning products are represented in Canada by Nelson Education, Ltd.

To learn more about Delmar, visit **www.cengage.com/delmar**

Purchase any of our products at your local college store or at our preferred online store **www.cengagebrain.com**

Printed in the United States of America
1 2 3 4 5 6 7 16 15 14 13 12

TABLE OF CONTENTS

Preface

Congratulations! By implementing the mentoring program found in this book, you are investing in all your CNAs, and especially the new ones just starting out in their caregiving careers. This mentoring program will offer them the support of a trained and experienced mentor to guide their way as they develop into quality health care professionals. Implementing this program will not only help you train and orient your new CNAs, it will also help knit them into the workplace community. If your facility invests the time and energy, this program will help you reduce your facility's CNA turnover, save you money, and build a more competent staff.

Conceptual Approach

Keep in mind that the book you're holding can be seen as a set of tools. What you do with these tools will determine the effectiveness of your program. We have tried to make it as easy as possible for you, but it's up to you and your facility to make it all come together. It is important to note that this program can and should be adapted and modified by you so it works best for your staff and your facility.

This book was written with the assumption that you, the reader, will be the "champion" of this program—that you, more than anyone else in your facility, will do what it takes to make this program a positive, lasting reality within your facility's work culture. Whether you take on the role of the program's "Training Instructor" and/or the "Mentors' Supervisor," this program will require your time and energy, particularly in the early stages as you are getting it established.

One of your early jobs will be to gain the buy-in and support of your facility. For this program to have a lasting, positive effect, and to be the agent of genuine change in your organization, your whole facility must be committed to its success—from the administrator to the CNAs.

Organization and Special Features

We've designed the curriculum in an easy-to-follow, scripted format so that your instructor can, with little preparation, start running the training class right away. We hope the instructor finds the curriculum a pleasure to use, and that he or she personalizes it over time.

Each of the six training modules is designed to take one hour of classroom instruction. For your students to receive maximum benefit from the training, we recommend classes be scheduled in a concentrated period of time, preferably within six or fewer consecutive weeks. One model that works is one 2-hour class each week for three consecutive weeks; each class will cover two modules.

In addition to brief lectures, each module includes various interactive exercises—such as question and answer sessions, group discussions, role playing, and brainstorming—to help make each session an enjoyable and memorable learning experience for your CNAs. The curriculum is designed for your instructor to engage students, and classes should be a true group learning experience where everyone's ideas and experiences play a part. For your classroom, try to use a designated area where the class won't be interrupted and your students can be comfortable and relaxed.

To make the teaching process easy for your instructor, each module is written in a script format that includes the following icons to indicate specific actions:

 SAY the following text to the class.

 READ the following passage or handout to the class.

 WRITE the following words for the whole class to see.

 DISTRIBUTE the following handout to the class.

 A HOT IDEA is a different or fun idea for a class exercise.

Note: Text that is intended only for the instructor appears in italic form and has no icon connected to it.

The Curriculum

The mentoring curriculum is the primary tool that you will use to train your mentors. Each of the six training modules is listed below along with its objectives:

Module 1—What Makes a Mentor?

Mentors will:

- Learn about their mentoring program
- Learn the definition of a mentor
- Understand their responsibilities as mentors
- Define the characteristics of an ideal caregiver

Module 2—Mentor as Teacher

Mentors will:

- Understand the characteristics of adult learners
- Discuss different learning styles
- Be shown how to evaluate the learning of the new CNA
- Appreciate the value of self-evaluation

Module 3—Mentor as Leader

Mentors will:

- Learn the definition of leadership
- Understand the two primary leadership styles
- Gain insights into their own leadership style
- Learn how to be leaders to their mentees

Module 4—Communication Skills

Mentors will:

- Gain an understanding of the basic elements of communication
- Understand and learn to practice active listening skills
- Understand and learn to practice giving good feedback

Module 5—Stress Management

Mentors will:

- Learn to identify and practice effective ways to reduce stress
- Understand and avoid unsuccessful ways of dealing with stress
- Learn to help their mentees cope with stress

- Recognize and check themselves for signs of stress

- Learn to reduce stress by managing time more effectively

Module 6—Your Job as a Mentor

Mentors will:

- Understand the duties and responsibilities of a mentor

- Learn what is expected of them during the new CNA's critical "break-in" period and beyond

- Be able to administer the evaluation forms

- Learn about providing ongoing support to the mentee

Module 7—A Booster Session for Mentors

Mentors will:

- Review key points from the earlier sessions of this program

- Identify problems and successes that have come up in their mentoring experience

- Brainstorm ideas for improving the mentoring program

New to this Edition

The second edition includes a new chapter that reinforces the effectiveness of the mentoring program through a "booster session." This new section includes organized feedback on the mentoring program, suggestions for problem resolution, and mutual support techniques.

New material on mentoring and person-centered care has been added, as well as a section specifically focusing on effective communication and mentoring documentation.

This new edition continues to offer handouts in the back of the text but also now includes these handouts on an Instructor Companion Website so that the materials can be more easily presented during training sessions.

The text has been thoroughly updated to reflect recent developments in the field.

Teaching Package for the Instructor

An Instructor Companion Website is now available and provides access to PowerPoint slides containing the handouts found at the back of the text, to facilitate use and presentation during training sessions.

About the Author

Karl Pillemer

Karl Pillemer, PhD, is a professor in the Human Development Department at Cornell University and director of the Cornell Institute for Translational Research on Aging. Throughout his career, Dr. Pillemer has conducted research and developed practical programs to improve the work life of nursing home staff. He is also a founder and consulting editor of *Nursing Assistant Monthly*, a newsletter that reaches thousands of certified nursing assistants each month.

Acknowledgments

Thank you to Rhoda Meador, Richard Hoffman, and Martin Schumacher, who contributed to the second edition of this text. I am grateful to two reviewers for their comments on the revision: Anna Ortigara, RN, MS, FAAN, Director of Communication and Outreach, THE GREEN HOUSE Project Tinley Park, Illinois; and Genevieve Gipson, Director, National Network of Career Nursing Assistants, Norton, Ohio.

This book is dedicated to those who do the hardest, most important job in America—nursing assistants. Were it not for their commitment, compassion, and skill, our elders would be without the loving care they deserve. Angels of mercy, guardians, healers, heroes—they are a shining example to us all.

Reviewers

Anna Ortigara, RN, MS, FAAN
Director of Communication and Outreach, THE GREEN HOUSE Project
Tinley Park, Illinois

Genevieve Gipson
Director, National Network of Career Nursing Assistants
Norton, Ohio

CNA
MENTORING
MADE
EASY

Introduction

What Is Mentoring?

The word *mentor* was first introduced in Homer's *Odyssey*. The goddess Athena disguised herself as Odysseus' old friend, Mentor, to advise Odysseus' son, Telemachus. Mentor/Athena acted as a teacher, nurturer, protector, advisor, and role model, whose goal it was to draw forth the young man's full potential.

In modern times, the word has come to mean any person who teaches, nurtures, protects, and advises another person. To grow and develop in our lives and careers, most of us need a mentor, or someone with experience who can help guide us along the way.

Good mentors offer their emotional and social support as well as skills and knowledge to their mentee. They share their life experiences and technical skills. They know how to listen, observe, and solve problems. In addition to being teachers and advisors, mentors serve as role models. By their example, they show their students what to do and how to act.

For any mentoring relationship to succeed, there must be understanding, respect, and trust on both sides. There needs to be a mutual willingness to share and a dedication to success.

Mentoring in Long-Term Care

Some jobs can be studied and then performed without a hitch, with only occasional brushing up on the necessary skills. Being a CNA and caring for people in long-term care facilities is not one of these jobs. In good caregiving, experience is crucial.

The alarmingly high turnover rates for CNAs attest to the fact that it is not an easy job. Some of the most promising new caregivers are discouraged early on, before they gain the experience necessary to handle the many emotional and interpersonal demands of the job. What can keep new CNAs on the job during those initial weeks while they begin to gain the crucial experience they need? In short, a good relationship with a qualified mentor. Mentoring is the essential link between training and quality caregiving.

The value of a peer mentoring program lasts long after the initial weeks of a CNA's employment. Besides helping to retain new staff, the program orients them to the expectations of the best of their peers and serves to cultivate the kind of teamwork and cohesiveness that results in quality care. It also helps them to be productive contributors sooner, as they see right from the start that their success is important to both their employer and their coworkers.

In short, there are many good reasons to invest time and energy into a mentoring program that will help you to:

- Recognize and reward experienced caregivers
- Assess the learning needs of new staff
- Standardize the orientation process
- Create an environment conducive to ongoing learning
- Provide support and guidance to new staff
- Teach the values of professional caregiving
- Accustom the new staff to the culture of the facility
- Ultimately, increase retention

Implementing Your Mentoring Program

In developing this mentoring program, we undertook a "best practice" review of successful mentoring programs throughout long-term care. The program you hold in your hands is a synthesis of the best qualities of a variety of mentoring programs from across the country.

The following pages lay out what you need to know and what decisions you need to make to start and run a successful program. This front section is followed by the curriculum, consisting of seven fully scripted, self-contained modules, which require little preparation time by your instructor. Each module follows a specific format and uses icons that signal specific actions for your instructor to take. Found within each module are references to student handouts that reinforce the curriculum and serve as a learning tool for your students; these handouts are located after the modules in numerical order. (Note: If your instructor uses PowerPoint, slides can be easily adapted from the handouts.)

It is important to note that this mentoring program consists of two distinct activities:

1. The mentor training period—when you prepare your students to become mentors. The training curriculum, contained in this book, is what your facility will use to conduct this training.

2. The mentoring process—when the mentor supports and teaches the new CNA, which occurs during the first month of the new CNA's employment. The mentor must first successfully complete the training period before acting as a mentor.

Eligibility Requirements

For the Mentor

Mentors should be chosen for their experience, maturity, clinical skills, commitment, and ability to be a positive role model for new caregivers. A mentor needs to be technically skilled, as well as a friendly and generous person. You will develop your own set of standards for applicants, but here are some specific suggestions.

To be eligible to become a mentor, a candidate should:

- Have worked in the facility for at least a year
- Have undergone no disciplinary action in the last year
- Fill out the application form completely
- Receive a recommendation from the Mentors' Supervisor
- Have an interview with the Director of Nursing or the Administrator.

Make sure your CNAs know about the program and what the eligibility requirements are. Make it clear who they can go to with questions and who will be handling the application process.

For the New CNA (or Mentees)

This mentoring program is meant to support new employees who are just beginning to work in your facility. If mentored from the first day on the job, they will gain the maximum benefits of the mentoring process.

Chances are that you will not be able to mentor every new CNA you hire, particularly in the early days of your program as it is getting established. In terms of priorities for choosing new CNAs to participate, we recommend you first select those nursing assistants who have recently been certified and are just starting out as caregivers; they, more than the experienced CNA, will benefit from a qualified mentor. The ideal is that every one of your new CNA hires, no matter how much experience they bring, could take part in your mentoring program.

Application Form

We suggest you develop a simple application form for qualified CNAs who would like to become mentors. A sample form has been provided in the back of this book (see Appendix 1) to serve as a guide for you.

Matching Mentors with New CNAs

How will you know how to match brand-new CNAs with your mentors? Instinct will be your guide in this decision. When you pair mentors with new CNAs, you should be looking to maximize learning while making sure the new CNA is comfortable and feels encouraged. If you see that the relationship is not working, change it. An unsuitable mentoring relationship will make both sides uncomfortable and will decrease the chances of the new CNA staying at your facility.

When choosing the new CNA/mentor pair, you may want to take their cultural or ethnic group into account. New caregivers often experience a lot of stress in the early days of a new job, and working with someone from a similar background may make this transition easier.

Setting Up Your Class

Choosing an Instructor

In choosing your instructor, first review the curriculum closely, and then ask yourself: Who would be the best choice to conduct this training? Is it your Staff Development Coordinator, or is it someone else? The ideal instructor is someone on staff who frequently comes in contact with CNAs, is a lively presenter who is good at drawing people out, and has a good understanding of the complexities of the caregiver's job.

Class Scheduling and Structure

As you schedule your class, you will need to consider how best to make the training sessions work in your facility. You may want to schedule the one-hour mentoring classes once a week, or you may want to combine the classes and teach several modules in two- or three-hour blocks. Whatever you choose, try to keep the overall training period relatively short, with no more than a six-week period from start to finish.

Plan to use a classroom or designated area where your students can be comfortable, can easily engage in the class exercises, and where residents or other staff will not interrupt.

Your class size should be small, ideally between six and eight students. A small class size makes it possible to create a level of comfort and intimacy impossible with a larger group, while allowing everyone to participate.

Evaluations

Evaluations forms are used to monitor the progress of both the mentor and her mentee and to point to areas that still need attention. Formal evaluations for both the new CNA and for the mentor will happen at the end of Week 1 and at the end of Month 1 with the use of supplied evaluation forms (see Handout 2-5 and Handout 2-6). The Mentors' Supervisor, or whoever is in charge of the program, should monitor the evaluation process continuously to make adjustments as needed.

For the New CNA (the Mentee)

Evaluations of the new CNA's progress are completed by the mentor at the end of Week 1 and at the end of Month 1. The mentor fills out the "New CNA Evaluation" (Handout 2-5) as a way to measure what the new CNA has mastered and what he or she needs improvement on. The mentor, the new CNA, and the Mentors' Supervisor should all sign this form, which should then be filed in the new CNA's employee file.

For the Mentor

Evaluations of the mentor are done by the new CNA (along with the Mentors' Supervisor, if you choose) at the end of Week 1 and at the end of Month 1. The new CNA fills out the "Mentor Evaluation" (Handout 2-6) as a way to measure the mentor's effectiveness, while giving the mentor some valuable feedback. The new CNA, mentor, and the Mentors' Supervisor should all sign this form, which should then be filed in the mentor's employee file.

Supervision of Mentors

As the mentors guide the new CNAs, they themselves will need someone to guide them. This person, whom we've referred to in this document as the "Mentors' Supervisor," should be the individual who is overseeing your mentoring program and who, if possible, is also the mentors' training instructor. This Mentors' Supervisor will need to continuously monitor the mentors' progress with the new CNAs and be there to offer assistance whenever necessary. This person should also be in charge of the evaluation process.

Recognition and Rewards

Being chosen as a mentor is an expression of confidence in the skill, experience, and professionalism of each CNA selected—and it is important that everyone in your facility is made aware of this, especially the mentors themselves. In terms of recognition, try to create an ongoing atmosphere of appreciation that emphasizes the importance of the mentor's role. This atmosphere is an important element for a successful program.

Another key element leading to the success of this program will be the mentors' perception that this is an opportunity both to improve the facility and to improve themselves by learning new skills and gaining recognition as a leader. Make sure that you take every opportunity to emphasize these mutually beneficial goals.

As for other rewards, it's your decision what your facility gives your mentors. Whatever you choose, make sure it's viewed as something significant by the mentors and the rest of the CNAs, and make sure people are aware of these rewards.

The following are recommendations on how to recognize and reward your mentors.

1. On acceptance into the mentoring program:

- The employee should receive a letter from the Mentors' Supervisor or Administrator. This letter should be sent to the CNA at home, offering congratulations on selection and extending the facility's gratitude for the CNA's promise to help, by participation in the program, in making your facility one of the best.

2. On completion of the training:

- Conduct a ceremony where mentors receive a graduation certificate and a pin designating their new mentor status. Have the Director of Nursing and Administrator attend, if possible.

- Display photos of your new mentors in a prominent place.

- Have a semi-annual luncheon for mentors to celebrate their contributions.

- Start a Mentor-of-the-Month program.

- Offer gift certificates to local theaters and restaurants.

3. After the mentoring period is completed:

- If a new mentored CNA remains on the job for three months, the mentor should receive a cash bonus of $100.

- If a new mentored CNA remains on the job for a full year, the mentor should receive an additional bonus of $200.

- Hold one or more follow-up sessions for mentors. In this manual, we provide the content for a "booster session" to reinforce the training principles and troubleshoot any problems that may emerge. Additional sessions are recommended to bring the mentors together to exchange experiences.

The Mentoring Period

After mentors have successfully completed the training, they are ready to begin the mentoring process. We have identified the formal mentoring period as the first month of a new CNA's employment in the facility. (Note: One month is the shortest period of time we recommend; in adapting this program to fit your facility, we strongly suggest you extend this mentoring period to two or more months, if possible.)

To make the mentoring work best, we have identified two key periods in the new CNA's work-life. The first is the "break-in period," the critical first week on the job. The second period is Weeks 2, 3, and 4, known as the period of "integration into the caregiving team." The mentor will provide guidance and support in different ways during these two periods.

Week 1: The "Break-in" Period

The first week on the job for a new CNA is critical. It is often during this time of first impressions that a new CNA decides whether the job is a "good fit." It is during this key "break-in" period when the CNA and the mentor, with the help and supervision of the Mentors' Supervisor, will spend the majority of their time together—as the new CNA moves from simply "shadowing" the mentor to beginning to take on his or her own resident care load. For a complete discussion of the "break-in" period, see Module 6, Topic #2. (Note: Mentors should have only one mentee during the "break-in" period unless their workload has been significantly reduced.)

Some of the duties of the mentor during this first week include the following:

- Give the new CNA a tour of the unit and facility.
- Introduce the new CNA to staff and residents.
- Be "shadowed" by the new CNA.
- Address the new CNA's problems and concerns.
- Give the new CNA limited resident care activities.
- Provide and supervise hands-on learning opportunities.
- Discuss daily assignments with the new CNA.
- Increase resident care activities for the new CNA.
- Offer feedback to the new CNA on a daily basis.
- Complete appropriate evaluation form.

To create the kind of relationship between mentor and new CNA that will result in excellent care and an ongoing commitment to the profession of caregiving, a brief period of intense help and support is usually not enough.

Weeks 2–4: Integration into the Caregiving Team

The second and final phase of the mentoring period takes place during Weeks 2 through 4 of the new CNA's employment. The role and level of activity of the mentor during this period of "integration into the caregiving team" will be determined at the end of the first week when the mentor and Mentors' Supervisor meet to evaluate the new CNA's progress. It is at this point that an assessment is made, using an evaluation form (see Handout 2-5), that will shape the next period of the mentoring relationship. For a complete discussion of this second period, see Module 6, Topic #3.

Depending on what is decided at the end of Week 1, the mentor's role in this second period may vary significantly, from one of almost daily interaction and assistance to one of periodic check-ins and relatively casual support for the new CNA. For this mentoring period to be successful, your facility will need to be flexible to accommodate both the mentor and the new CNA. Here is a list of the possible responsibilities of the mentor during this period:

- Meet with the new CNA on a regular, scheduled basis to offer support, feedback, and to address any concerns or problems.

- Provide and supervise hands-on learning opportunities.

- Offer additional caregiving and clinical expertise.

- Act as ongoing social support.

- Intercede with others on the new CNA's behalf, if necessary.

- Continue to increase the caregiving assignments, as appropriate, until the new CNA has a full resident care load.

- Complete and turn in evaluation forms.

After the Mentoring Period

The end of the first month marks the conclusion of the formal mentoring arrangement. If the mentor and the Mentors' Supervisor both feel that the new CNA has gained full independence and is ready to "go out on his or her own," then they should take a moment to congratulate each other as well as their new caregiver.

Ongoing Support, Direction, and Advice

If, however, the mentor or the Mentors' Supervisor feels that the CNA could benefit from the mentor relationship continuing in some capacity, then it should if at all possible. If the new CNA stills needs ongoing support, or direction, or advice from the mentor, then it will benefit your facility to make the necessary arrangements.

In this same spirit, if it is possible within your facility, you should encourage all participants in this program to continue meeting and working together, as mentors and mentees, beyond the arbitrary period of one month. Your facility will be the better for it.

While no program can mandate friendships, it can help to create advisors and allies to new CNAs during their often difficult adjustment to work in the nursing home. We hope that your new CNAs and your mentors will forge professional and personal bonds that continue well after the formal mentoring process is over.

Eight Easy Steps for Launching Your Program

Now that you know the benefits of this mentoring program and how it works, you're ready to launch your own program. Begin with these eight easy steps.

Step 1. Read this book.

This book is where you start. Use it as you would an owner's manual, and refer back to it as needed. Remember: You will need to adjust and adapt this program so it works best for your staff and your facility.

Step 2. Promote the program.

Let everyone in your facility know about the program: what it is and why it's important. Discuss the program with your colleagues on the nursing and administrative staff. They can serve as valuable allies and supporters when they understand the real benefits of the program.

Step 3. Choose your training instructor.

Who is the best person to run the mentor training? Your selection here is very important, as the instructor's approach and comfort level with the CNAs will have a major impact on the success of the program.

Step 4. Recruit and select your mentors.

The success of your program will partly depend on the quality of your mentors. You will want to recruit CNAs who embody the highest standards of caregiving and whose behavior and attitude will serve as an exemplary model for your future employees. Determine appropriate eligibility requirements, prepare an application form (see example provided), and begin the selection process.

Step 5. Review and customize the training modules.

Have your instructor familiarize himself or herself with the content so that the instructor can personalize it as much as possible. The curriculum pages have room on which to write speaker notes. One simple way to personalize is to add examples and names from your facility.

Step 6. Determine class logistics.

Allow a little time to select the right schedule and location for the mentoring classes. Try to accommodate as many people's schedules as possible. Choose a classroom site that will help to ensure that the training is private and comfortable for all.

Step 7. Conduct the mentor training.

Once the logistics have been determined, make sure that the training classes happen as planned. The integrity of the program and the enthusiasm of its participants will be jeopardized if the classes don't occur as scheduled. Ideally, the classes are something that everyone, from student to instructor, plans for and looks forward to.

Step 8. Start the mentoring process.

Once the training is completed, you're ready to begin the mentoring process. Now, each time you hire a new CNA, match the new CNA up with one of your new mentors. You have set the stage for building an excellent and stable caregiving staff. Congratulations!

Launching and Running Your Mentoring Program

SAMPLE TIMELINE — 12-WEEK PERIOD

1	2	3	4	5	6	7	8	9	10	11	12

WEEK 1 — Read *CNA Mentoring Made Easy.*

WEEKS 2 - 12 — Promote the program on an ongoing basis.
Explain to facility stakeholders what mentoring is and why it's important.

WEEKS 3, 4 — Choose your training instructor.

WEEKS 4, 5, 6 — Recruit and select your mentors. Determine eligibility requirements and solicit applications.

WEEKS 4, 5, 6 — Determine class logistics.

WEEKS 6, 7, 8 — Conduct mentor training: teach two modules per week, for three consecutive weeks.

WEEK 9 — Begin mentoring process: one week "Break-in" period.

WEEK 10, 11, 12 — Complete mentoring process: three week "Integration into the Caregiving Team" period.

Frequently Asked Questions

What are the specific duties and responsibilities of a mentor?
See Module 6 and Handouts 6-2, 6-3, 6-4, 6-5, and 6-6.

Should I pay my CNAs for the time they are in the mentoring classes?
Mentors should be paid for their time and at their normal rate during the mentoring classes. Payment for the learning process will add legitimacy to your program and help motivate mentors to stay involved.

Should new CNAs be paid during the first week while they are mentees?
Yes, they should be paid a regular salary during this first week. Serving as mentees should be viewed as a necessary part of their training.

Do I need to work this program into our existing orientation?
This mentoring program will work best if it is integrated into your regular orientation activities. You will want to consider how to plan and schedule both events so that they reinforce and enhance one another.

Should the mentors continue meeting after their training classes are over?
You should consider a regular monthly group meeting for all the mentors in your facility to provide additional training and program updates. Some kind of periodic forum for all your mentors makes good sense: It helps to reinforce their identity as mentors while giving them an opportunity to discuss with their peers any concerns or challenges they might be facing.

Tips and Techniques for the Instructor

Conducting Great Role Plays

Role plays offer an opportunity for mentor trainees to "put themselves in the shoes" of new CNAs and to practice new skills in a supportive atmosphere. Role plays can also enliven the training, stimulate discussion, and show participants different ways of handling a situation.

Here are some guidelines for conducting good role plays along with a few tips for handling any difficulties that might arise:

- Introduce the role play with enthusiasm. Participants will pick up on your attitudes, so try to be positive.

- Briefly explain the benefits of role playing. Learners need to know why they are participating.

- Emphasize that there are no "right" or "wrong" ways to role play.

- Ask for volunteers. Don't force anyone to role play.

- If people are slow to fill the roles, conduct a small-group role play, in which people participate in groups of six or less.

- If participants are hesitant to volunteer, role play a part yourself.

- Remember to use your sense of humor and have fun!

Leading Case Study Discussions

The mentor training curriculum uses case studies as a teaching tool. These stories and anecdotes enhance learning by taking abstract concepts and making them concrete. Case studies can bring examples to life by providing familiar details from the work setting. They can help participants think in new ways about common challenges that they might have encountered.

To make case studies effective, it's important for the instructor to keep a few guidelines in mind:

- Ask questions about the case studies to stimulate discussion.

- Encourage participants to react by affirming their comments.

- Keep the discussion open and nonjudgmental.

Final Tips for the Instructor

On a final note, before your first training class begins, here are several suggestions we hope your instructor will take to heart:

DON'T—set your expectations too high in the beginning.

DON'T—be too rigid in following the curriculum. If an exercise or a role play isn't working, move on to something else.

DON'T—read directly from the script. This is boring for both you and your class.

DON'T—forget about the importance of the training environment. Try to find a comfortable setting for your class and offer refreshments, if possible.

DON'T—assume that because a participant is quiet, he or she is not learning anything; some people may have trouble speaking up but are still learning.

DO—involve your administrator in the program from the very beginning, and keep him or her updated on the progress.

DO—rehearse the exercises and role plays before you teach the class.

DO—put the lectures in your own words.

DO—feel free to modify the case studies and role plays to include situations that are more appropriate to your facility.

DO—set a relaxed and friendly tone in the classroom. This is not a place where people will be judged harshly; it is a group learning experience, where a participant's stories and experiences should play an integral part.

DO—have fun!

CNA
MENTORING
MADE
EASY

Program Curriculum

MODULE 1

What Makes a Mentor?

Objectives of this Module

Mentors will:

- Learn about their mentoring program
- Learn the definition of a mentor
- Understand their responsibilities as mentors
- Define the characteristics of an ideal caregiver

Introduction

For The Instructor Only

Take a moment before you facilitate the first session to reflect on the perspective of the participants in your group. Many of them may be wondering: "Why am I here? What makes me special enough to be chosen for a mentoring program? How is this program going to work?"

Your first goal, as an instructor, will be to build the self-confidence of the mentors. They have come to this training with many years of rich experience as professional care-givers. Make sure that they know they have been chosen for this program because they are some of the best caregivers in your facility. They have been chosen for their fine qualities as teachers, guides, and mentors. They deserve to be recognized and praised for their hard work, dedication, and desire to go beyond their normal duties to help new CNAs.

This first module will give you an overview of mentoring, ex-plain what a mentor is, what traits a good mentor has, and what different responsibilities belong to a mentor.

TOPIC #1

What Is a Mentor?

Introduce yourself and take a few minutes to help the group members get to know each other. Ask them to share:

- *Their name*

- *How long they've worked as a CNA*

- *A few words about themselves and why they chose to work with elders*

This may be harder for caregivers who have been there for many years. Make sure you encourage them with positive feedback about the wealth of their experience. Write on the board how many years each person has been a CNA.

 To begin, SAY:

It looks like we have a lot of experience in this room! Besides using this experience in your jobs as excellent CNAs, what else can you do with it? If I were a resident, I would feel safe in the hands of such experienced caregivers. And if I were a new CNA, I would want to benefit from all that experience.

This program was created so you could pass on that experience to new CNAs. When some one has as much experience as you, we often call that person an expert. This program aims to help you pass this expert knowledge on to our new CNAs. We hope that, in time, the residents in the new CNA's care will begin receiving the same excellent care as your residents.

You are all in this mentoring program because you have proven to be exceptional caregivers. You have been chosen for your personal character as well as your experience. Our facility believes we need more caregivers just like you. We wish all new CNAs could be as good as you from the start.

Since this is impossible—seeing the years of experience that you have—we are going to work with you to pass on your knowledge to new CNAs. In working to become mentors, you contribute to some very important goals:

- Building an excellent caregiving staff

- Ensuring that our residents receive the highest possible quality of care

- Making excellent care the standard in this facility

So, what makes a mentor?

 WRITE on the board:

Mentor:

A person who takes a special interest in helping someone else learn, develop, and succeed.

 DISTRIBUTE Handout 1-1: Definition of Mentor.

 Then SAY:

Whenever we start in a new situation, it helps to have a more experienced person—whether a coworker or a friend— advise us. It's reassuring to have someone who has been down that path before guide us along our own path.

Mentors impart more than their caregiving and clinical skills to new CNAs. They also give emotional and social support. Seasoned CNAs who become mentors know that a CNA must be a compassionate, caring person, as well as clinically and technically skilled.

What is needed for a mentoring relationship to succeed? There must be understanding, respect, and trust on both sides. The mentor's part of the bargain begins with accepting and respecting the mentee. A successful mentor has good listening, problem-solving, and observation skills. Successful mentors are also willing to share their technical skills, as well as their life experiences. Most importantly, they establish an environment in which the person they mentor has every opportunity to succeed.

TOPIC #2

The Mentor

Read over the following handout with the class. Explain that this handout outlines the groundwork for the mentoring program. The training they will receive in this program will help them fulfill these responsibilities.

 DISTRIBUTE Handout 1-2: Overview of the Mentor's Job.

 After reviewing the handout, SAY:

There are three basic functions of a mentor—teacher, role model, and supporter. Let's look at Handout 1-2 again and match the mentor's responsibilities to the three functions listed on Handout 1-3. Which responsibilities belong to which function? Are there any that fit into more than one function?

DISTRIBUTE Handout 1-3: The Three Functions of a Mentor.

Brainstorm with the class members, writing their answers on the board.

 Now SAY:

These three basic functions are equally important in turning your mentee into an ideal CNA, one who may become as good a CNA as you. Now that we've given the ingredients for a good mentor, let's see what goes into a good caregiver. Let's try an exercise to see what your recipe for a perfect caregiver is.

 WRITE on the board:

- Technical skills
- Resident care skills
- Communication skills
- Customer service skills
- Personal qualities

Break the class into smaller groups of three or four people. Read the directions below, having each group write its answers on a piece of paper. After about 15 minutes, the groups should present their "recipes."

 To conclude, SAY:

A successful recipe depends on the right combination of ingredients. For it to work, it has to have the right amount of each ingredient and be prepared in a certain way. A great caregiver is also made up of a combination of skills and qualities that you can help "prepare."

As master chefs, you will come up with many recipes for the ideal caregiver. Follow these steps to create your recipe.

- Use the categories listed on the board to come up with your ingredients.

- You may even want to add some additional ingredients that you think of on your own.

- How much of each will be required? Can you assign a percentage to each ingredient?

- How can you help these ingredients work best together?

Good luck on your new creations and—bon appetit!

After the groups make their presentations, have the participants share and discuss their recipes.

MODULE 2

Mentor as Teacher

Objectives of this Module

Mentors will:

- Understand the characteristics of adult learners
- Discuss different learning styles
- Learn how to evaluate the learning of the new CNA
- Appreciate the value of self-evaluation

TOPIC #1

How Adults Learn

 To begin, SAY:

Think back to when you were in school. You may have thought a pencil, some paper, and simply showing up were enough to learn. For adult learners, however, it's more complex than that. Research shows that adults learn differently than children do.

Some of the things that we know about how adults learn are:

1. Adult learners are diverse. They vary among ages, abilities, experiences, cultural backgrounds, and goals.

2. They bring a wide range of personal experiences that are valuable resources.

3. Adult learners want to relate what they learn to their daily lives. They need to know how the new knowledge will be useful to them.

4. They prefer to have some control over their learning. It is important to give them opportunities to have some direction over how and what they need to know.

5. The adult learners' attitudes about the learning experience are very important. They may have bad feelings about some negative experiences in school. It is very important to give them lots of positive feedback.

Above all, learning is a matter of attitude. Learners must be able to admit they don't know everything, be able to ask someone to teach them what they don't know, and have enough confidence to try new things. Becoming a good learner requires learning, in other words. This may sound confusing, but let's take it one step at a time. Your first step should be taking responsibility for your learning.

Remember the three functions of a mentor? One role you will play as a mentor is teacher. You're probably thinking, *Me? A teacher?* Obviously, you have already exhibited teaching potential, since you're in this mentoring program. To become a true teacher, you must first understand how people learn. Let's begin by defining what it means to learn.

 WRITE on the board:

Learning:

To acquire knowledge of a subject or skill as a result of study, experience, or instruction.

 DISTRIBUTE Handout 2-1: Definition of Learning.

 Now SAY:

This definition of learning is general. The way people learn is much more complex. By the time we reach adulthood, everyone learns in a different way. We find a way to learn that works the best for us by trial and error. Adults often combine a variety of learning styles but rely on the one they find most comfortable. As a student or as a teacher, it helps to know what your learning style is.

 DISTRIBUTE Handout 2-2: The Four Types of Learners.

 As you DISTRIBUTE the handout, SAY:

When we learn, we combine our brains, eyes, ears, and hands in our own unique way. Our "learning style" is the combination we feel most comfortable with and prefer.

A Hot Idea

What is your learning style?

Review Handout 2-2. Conduct a discussion with the class, using the following steps:

1. Have each person try to remember a time when he or she successfully learned something specific. It can be anything— the first time they properly transferred a resident, when they first changed a tire, when they baked a cake.

2. Ask them to describe how they learned it. What was the process?

3. Have the rest of the class try to guess what the teller's learning style is.

4. Ask the teller if he or she agrees with the class's opinion. The tellers may be surprised at the difference between what they thought and what the class says.

 Now WRITE on the board:

Teaching:

To show someone the way: to direct or guide. To communicate knowledge.

 DISTRIBUTE Handout 2-3: Definition of Teaching.

Then SAY:

While people are in school, they don't usually pay attention to how their teachers present the material. They are more interested in the content of the material, in memorizing and learning it the best they can. As teachers-in-training, you will need to think about your presentation. You will have to decide how to best present your material and how to tailor it to the person you're teaching.

Before you can decide how to teach material to a certain person, though, you've got to choose which material to teach. You wouldn't want to teach a new CNA how to feed a particular resident if they already know how; but you also wouldn't want to assume they know how to document ADLs if they don't. You should prepare to teach by first assessing the new CNA's learning needs.

In the early days, when the new CNA is "shadowing" you, there will be many questions on both sides. You should be getting to know each other as coworkers and as people. As you would expect, most of their questions will be about the facility, the residents, procedures, and such. You should be asking questions to find out what the new CNA needs to learn the most and how she can learn it best. What questions could you ask a new CNA?

Conduct a discussion about questions to ask new CNAs. Have the class remember the earlier exercise when they recounted successful learning stories. Tell them that asking new CNAs to do this exercise may help them as teachers. It can clue them in to that person's learning style.

 WRITE the ideas on the board. Discuss each one.

TOPIC #2

Evaluating Learning

 To begin, SAY:

As you ask the new CNA questions about herself or himself, you are starting the evaluation process. As you continue to instruct the CNA, you will assess the CNA's needs in two important ways. The first is through what the CNA tells you his or her needs are. The second is through deeds; the CNA's performance will show you where he or she still needs help and what he or she has mastered. In evaluating strengths and weaknesses, you will adjust your focus and instruction accordingly. It will be equally important to praise accomplishments and encourage the CNA to work on improving performance.

 WRITE on the board:

Evaluate:

To ascertain or fix the value or worth of.

To examine or judge carefully.

 DISTRIBUTE Handout 2-4: Definition of Evaluate.

 To continue, SAY:

Let's have a look at one of the primary evaluation tools you will be using.

 DISTRIBUTE Handout 2-5: New CNA Evaluation.

A Hot Idea

For a brainstorming session:

Have the class review Handout 2-5, then start a brainstorm. Have them consider: When we use this evaluation form, what will it tell us? What kinds of questions might one have on completing the form? Write their answers on the board. These could include:

- What skills has the new CNA mastered?
- What does the new CNA need help with?
- What things are the hardest for the new CNA?
- What do you still need to work on as the new CNA's mentor?

Now SAY:

This form is the primary evaluation tool you will be using. It will be filled in, signed, and turned in to your supervisor two times: at the end of the first week of the new CNA's hire and at the end of the first month. In addition to letting your supervisor and your facility know how things are going, it's a way for you to monitor the progress of the CNA, as well as your own progress as a mentor.

To continue, SAY:

Remember, our ultimate goal is to see every new CNA succeed. Evaluations will show you what improvements are needed for them to succeed. When giving your feedback after the evaluations, keep in mind that constructive criticism is usually taken better with a little praise thrown in. People are more receptive to criticism when they don't feel they're under attack.

Can you remember how it felt when you were a new CNA and there were a lot of new things to learn? Put yourself in the shoes of the new CNA. Encourage him or her by emphasizing the progress he or she is making, as well as pointing out the areas that need work. Be clear, supportive, and positive about changes that need to occur.

As you see on the evaluation form, both you and your supervisor are required to sign the form, as well as the new CNA. For this program to be successful, there must be a partnership between mentors and their supervisor. You will be our eyes and ears to see how the new CNA is doing. Your supervisor will be there to support you, help you teach the new CNA, and help you resolve any problems that might come up.

 DISTRIBUTE Handout 2-6: Mentor Evaluation.

 To conclude, SAY:

Evaluations are useful for the new CNA as a way of highlighting strengths and weaknesses. They can be just as useful for you to see what your strengths and weaknesses are as a mentor. To see how you are doing as a mentor, we will have new CNAs fill out evaluations similar to the ones you will do for them. The purpose is not to test you, but to check in on how you're doing and if there's any room for improvement. You will have a copy of the mentor evaluation, so you can check on your own progress.

Your experience as a mentor is an opportunity to continue to develop as a professional caregiver and teacher. You were chosen to be a mentor because of your excellence as a CNA and your interpersonal skills with other people. The evaluation is a good opportunity to get new information that can help you grow and improve your skills even more.

Like the new CNA evaluations, your evaluations will be done two times: at the end of the first week and at the end of the first month. They will also be signed by you, the new caregiver, and your supervisor. For the program to truly succeed, to create an exceptional caregiving staff, we must all work together, which includes giving each other constant feedback.

MODULE 3

Mentor as Leader

Objectives of this Module

Mentors will:

- Learn the definition of leadership
- Understand the two primary leadership styles
- Gain insights into their own leadership style
- Learn how to be leaders to their mentees

TOPIC #1

What Is Leadership?

 To begin, SAY:

You are a leader, whether you realize it or not. Along with your caregiving skills and teaching ability, this is one of the reasons you were selected for this mentoring program. You are leading new CNAs along the path to excellence. Remember, you are their leader and guide in the nursing home, as well as the field of long-term care.

Have a class discussion about leadership. On the board, come up with a list of good leadership qualities and some examples of good leaders. Ask questions such as the following:

- *What does a leader do?*
- *What qualities does a leader have?*
- *Can you think of someone who has these qualities?*

 After the discussion, SAY:

Keep in mind: A leader's success is measured by the success of those he or she leads. Now compare your answers to those on this next handout.

 DISTRIBUTE Handout 3-1: A Leader Is . . .

 To continue, SAY:

One of the reasons we chose you for this program is your leadership ability. Each of you already has and uses these leadership skills. Let's talk about the four skills listed on the handout and how they relate to your work.

Discuss the ways experienced CNAs have acquired the skills listed in Handout 3-1 in their work. Ask the following questions:

- *What decisions do you make?*
- *What problems do you solve?*
- *How have you learned to organize your work?*
- *How does quality care depend on setting the right priorities?*

Have them write out their answers, then read them aloud to the class. Give positive reinforcement and emphasize that these leadership skills have made their facility a better place.

After the discussion has wound down,

 WRITE on the board:

Role Model:

Person on whom others model themselves.

 DISTRIBUTE Handout 3-2: Definition of a Role Model.

 Now SAY:

One of the functions of a leader is being a role model. Whether a new CNA knows it or not, he or she is using you as a model caregiver. This modeling comes partly from what you teach and partly from what the CNA picks up from your actions and attitude.

Ideally, every new CNA we hire would have many of the same qualities that make you such excellent caregivers. New CNAs can learn to be the kind of effective professional that you have become by doing the following things:

- Observing you
- Learning from you
- Using you as a guide

As a professional CNA, one of your most important contributions is the certain set of values that you bring to your job. These values shape your beliefs and your actions that demonstrate to the world what you think matters the most. You have developed these values through your life experiences over the years.

These values include:

 WRITE the following on the board:

- <u>Taking pride in your work</u>
- <u>Being a dependable coworker</u>
- <u>Being open to others' opinions</u>

 ASK the group:

- What other values would you add to this list?
- How would you practice or demonstrate these values?
- How do these values make you a better caregiver?

Discuss and reflect on the answers.

 To continue, SAY:

Being a truly good role model means many things:

- Practicing what you preach
- Letting your values as a caregiver shine through
- Showing your best caregiving skills
- Giving the new CNA every reason to look up to you
- Leading by example

TOPIC #2

Leadership Styles

 To begin, SAY:

There are many different styles of leaders, each with their own set of characteristics or traits. On one extreme, you have the "facilitative" or democratic leader who acts as a team leader, collaborating and delegating as much as possible. On the other extreme, you have the "directive" or autocratic leader who makes all the major decisions and tells others what to do.

Most effective leaders fall somewhere in between these two extremes, incorporating traits from one or both of these two opposing styles. The point is, no one style works for all people or in all situations.

To begin to understand different leadership styles, let's start by looking at these two primary leadership styles.

 DISTRIBUTE Handout 3-3: Two Primary Leadership Styles.

After discussing the handout and making sure everyone understands the traits of the two leadership styles, organize the following brainstorming session.

A Hot Idea

For a brainstorming session:

(Use Handouts 3-3, 3-4, 3-5, 3-6, and 3-7 for this session.)

Have the class break up into four groups. Give each group one of the scenarios found in Handouts 3-4 through 3-7 along with a copy of Handout 3-3 and let them decide which specific leadership traits (from Handout 3-3) would be most effective in each situation. After 10 to 15 minutes, have each group present its scenario to the class, including which specific traits group members chose and why.

 To conclude, SAY:

Leadership is something that needs constant practice. It involves not only what you say but also what you do. As you begin your new role, remember that leaders need other leaders. A lack of support and understanding can hurt even the best leaders. Remember that you are not alone. There are other people in this facility who can support you, and act as a role model for you, when you need it.

In my role as instructor, I'm here to help you. Use me as a resource to ask questions, voice concerns, or test ideas.

Your classmates can also be a resource for you. Practice using each other for support, guidance, and advice. When you have moments of uncertainty, learn to lean on one another. Good leaders know when they need help and where they can get it.

MODULE 4

Communication Skills

Mentors will:

- Gain an understanding of the basic elements of communication
- Understand and learn to practice active listening skills
- Understand and learn to practice giving good feedback
- Consider person-centered care principles when communicating with residents

TOPIC #1

What Is Communication?

 To begin, SAY:

As we all know, communication in the nursing home can be challenging. Often people in a nursing home, no matter what their role, experience stress. And when we are stressed, we don't communicate as effectively.

New CNAs often experience stress more acutely than other CNAs. If they are too stressed, their ability to learn suffers. They want to learn the new routines, master all the skills, and fit in all at the same time. They may be unsure about how to do something but are too afraid to ask for help. This could be even harder if they don't feel they can communicate with you as their mentor.

How can you make communication with the new CNA go more smoothly? How can you, as the mentor, model good communication skills? First, we need to examine what communication means.

 DISTRIBUTE Handout 4-1: The Elements of Communication.

 Then SAY:

Though you may not have thought of it this way before, the message is a vital part of communication. Conflicts are not usually about the sender or the receiver, though they often feel that way; they're usually about the message itself. Often, there is a misunderstanding about the message. The purpose of effective communication is to have the same message understood by both sender and receiver.

Remember that old game "Telephone," where everyone would sit in a circle and whisper a message from person to person? Let's give it a try for old times' sake.

A Hot Idea

For a game of "Telephone":

Have the class sit in a circle. Whisper one of the following messages to the first person, have that person whisper it to the person next to him or her, and so on until it goes around the circle. Tell them to repeat it exactly as they hear it.

1. "Sandra slipped on the ice outside her house and broke her ankle last Wednesday."

2. "Sandra's doctor told her not to walk on her broken ankle for the next two weeks."

3. "Mary will cover Sandra's Thursday shift and Karen will work for her on Friday."

Have the last person say the message aloud and write it on the board. Then write the original message on the board. How different is the final message from the one you initially whispered?

 To continue, SAY:

It may seem silly, but this game illustrates how confused a message can get when it's passed along between people. People listen differently, bringing their own personality and expectations to how they interpret messages.

How can we improve communication? What can we do to make sure messages are understood accurately? One way is called "active listening"—a skill all great communicators have.

TOPIC #2

Active Listening

 To begin, SAY:

You may think, *Active listening? If I'm listening, I'm listening.* If you are not actively paying attention to a message that someone is trying to communicate, then you are just hearing. Hearing is very different from active listening. To hear is to passively perceive sounds with the ear. To really listen is to try to understand what it being said. When you listen, you try to understand what the sender is both feeling and saying.

Why do we have only one mouth and two ears? Some might say it's so we can listen twice as hard as we talk. Others would say because listening is twice as hard as talking. In your role as mentor, you'll find that listening well is critical, and to do this, you need to engage in active listening.

 WRITE on the board:

Active Listening:

Understanding what the sender of
a message is thinking and feeling.

 DISTRIBUTE Handout 4-2: Definition of Active Listening.

 To continue, SAY:

It's helpful to remember the following key points about active listening:

- An active listener tries to understand both what the message means and what the sender feels.

- After the sender has communicated their message, the receiver, or active listener, should repeat the message back to make sure it has been understood.

- Then, before the receiver reacts to the message, the sender can clarify the message if needed.

- The receiver must feed back only the message he or she has heard, without adding personal feelings to it.

- When this happens, the sender feels he or she is being listened to and understood, and will ultimately be more receptive to how the receiver then reacts to the message.

Active listening isn't easy. It's something that needs to be learned and practiced. Here are some guidelines that will help you.

 DISTRIBUTE Handout 4-3: Guidelines for Active Listening.

 After reviewing the handout, SAY:

How can you be sure that the message the sender sends is the same one the receiver gets, since each receiver also becomes a sender?

Active listening skills can help ensure that the sender and the receiver are on the same page. As I said earlier, communication is made up of a sender, a message, and a receiver. I also said that conflict usually happens because the sender and receiver understand the message differently. Communication is more effective when we actively listen to a message and verify what has been said.

As a mentor, you will take on many roles—guide, teacher, leader. Now, who wants to try on another one—one of actor?

A Hot Idea

For a role play:

Follow these steps:

1. Ask two class members to demonstrate active listening.

2. One person should tell a story or personal anecdote with a complex plot.

3. The other person should listen as best he or she can, then ask questions to help clarify the story.

4. Allow the storyteller a few minutes to come up with a story before you begin.

5. Have two or three pairs of people repeat the exercise.

If your students choose not to come up with one of their own stories, then use one of the following:

- Margaret was a victim of resident aggression in her first week as a CNA. Mrs. Green, a resident with dementia, threw her dinner tray at Margaret when she tried to feed her. Since you're Margaret's mentor, she has come to you crying and saying she never wants to deal with Mrs. Green again.

- Sally, a new CNA, tells her mentor that she's not sure she's "cut out for this work" and that she has been depressed about her new job. Seeing the frail residents makes her so upset that she's not sure she wants to be a CNA.

After a few pairs have done their role plays, have the class identify and discuss which active listening and communication skills were used. Ask for suggestions about what additional skills should have been incorporated.

TOPIC #3

Feedback

 To begin, SAY:

Feedback is an important part of active listening. Let's talk about feedback and how to use it effectively. What makes good feedback?

 DISTRIBUTE Handout 4-4: Tips for Good Feedback.

 WRITE on the board:

Focus on the behavior, not the person.

 Now SAY:

Talk about what a person does, rather than about their personality. For example, being called "bossy" is not as effective as being told, "You were telling other CNAs to answer all the call lights, saying that you were too busy to do it." Describing a behavior allows for the possibility of change; calling someone a name is insulting and suggests that the person cannot change.

 WRITE on the board:

Be specific rather than general.

 SAY:

Be clear and concise when describing the problem behavior as well as the solutions. Instead of saying someone is "sloppy," say, "I know you're busy, but you left Mrs. Lewis's clothes scattered on her floor." Don't try to guess or assume what a person means by what they say or do. You also need to commit to hearing the other person's perspective. Ask clarifying questions to help them explain their actions.

WRITE on the board:

Be supportive.

 Now SAY:

Feedback should help rather than hurt. It takes the receiver's and sender's needs into account. Feedback used to gain power over another person or make the person feel bad is not good feedback, or good mentoring.

 WRITE on the board:

Emphasize what's possible and beneficial.

 SAY:

Only give as much information as the speaker can handle and benefit from. If a person is overloaded with feedback, it may not be useful. If the problem is beyond the speaker's control or due to a physical characteristic, he or she will only become more frustrated.

 WRITE on the board:

Take timing into account.

 SAY:

Immediate feedback is usually the most useful. The feedback should be well timed and should take into account the person's readiness to hear it. Since feedback can produce emotional reactions, be sensitive to the time and place it is given.

 WRITE on the board:

Invite feedback on the feedback.

Now SAY:

As a good active listener, you know it's good to rephrase what someone has said to make sure you understand him or her. Have the new CNA do this with your feedback to make sure he or she understands it. Sometimes the fragile or anxious state of the new CNA can cause misunderstandings that could be cleared up with good communication.

Next, try the following exercise.

 ## A Hot Idea

For an exercise in problem solving:

Each class member should try to solve the problem presented in the following two scenarios. First, read scenario 1 out loud. After giving class members time to think, write down their answers on the board and have a discussion about them. Do the same thing for scenario 2.

SCENARIO 1

1. Betty, a new CNA whom you are mentoring, speaks to an upset family member in an unpleasant, curt manner. She has been speaking to coworkers and residents in the same way. Though she is doing her tasks correctly and in a timely manner, her attitude has been a definite problem. What kind of feedback would you give to this new CNA?

SCENARIO 2

2. You have been selected to mentor Jane, a new CNA on your unit. She seems to be a hard worker, but you notice that she is very negative and pessimistic in discussions with coworkers. One day you need to give her some feedback on a mistake that she made when trying to lift a resident. Jane is so busy trying to deny that she lifted the resident incorrectly, she won't listen to you describe the correct way to do it. How would you get Jane to stop and listen?

TOPIC #4

A Person-Centered Approach to Communicating with Residents

 To begin, SAY:

A person who moves into a nursing home experiences more than a move to a new place. For many, the recent past has been very painful and full of losses. They may have recently suffered the loss of a spouse or other close companion. They may have had to give up valuable possessions, even their homes, to make the care they need possible. Being admitted to a nursing facility may seem like the biggest loss of all—the loss of independence. For some, it is what they have feared most.

Some residents can feel vulnerable, fearful, disoriented, and may be feeling abandoned and hopeless. How can new CNAs, as the people who will have the most contact with residents, help to make this their home, where they feel respected, comfortable, and as fulfilled as possible?

For residents to feel truly at home, a new CNA has to get to know the person, this unique individual before them. One of the most important aspects of communicating with residents is to see the whole person and to understand that person's history and personality. And that's where the idea of *person-centered care* comes in.

 WRITE on the board:

What are some things a CNA could learn about a resident that would be helpful in understanding him or her?

List the answers from the group on the board. If the following are not mentioned, you can add them to the list:

What does the resident value?

What is the resident afraid of?

What did the resident do for a living?

Is the resident married? Does he or she have children? Other close family members?

How involved are the family members?

Is religion important to the resident?

What does the resident like to do?

Discuss the answers and why the information might be important in understanding and communicating with the resident.

 Now SAY:

It's exactly these kinds of things that make up person-centered care. Your role as a mentor includes helping new CNAs to relate to the whole person, understanding his or her wishes and needs, and thinking up creative solutions for how to meet them.

The model of *person-centered care* is being used in more and more nursing homes. It's an active approach to thinking about and responding to working with residents in a new way. It can dramatically improve the quality of life for residents. Practiced regularly and consistently, person-centered care can improve how the new CNAs work with residents and their families.

You as a mentor can help new employees think in terms of person-centered care. It can help them find solutions to residents' problems and to look at nursing home life in a new way.

We can't cover the whole topic of person-centered care in this session, but there's one principle that is especially important for helping CNAs communicate with, and about, residents.

 WRITE on the board:

All behavior has meaning.

Ask the group what they think this might mean and discuss.

Then ask specifically: What might this mean when a CNA is caring for a resident with dementia?

 Now SAY:

This concept is a cornerstone of person-centered care. For example, the behavior of a resident with dementia may seem strange and chaotic to a new CNA. But the resident's behavior is an attempt to communicate a need, a wish, a feeling. Engaged in a continual effort to look to the *meaning* behind the behavior, the person-centered approach leads us to rethink our interpretations of "problem behaviors."

The model is based on the technique of putting yourself in the resident's shoes, getting "into his or her skin," looking at the world through the resident's eyes. Sounds easy, but it takes some practice. In your interactions with new CNAs, you can encourage them to really try to understand who the residents are, their life histories, and who they were before they developed the health problems that led them to the nursing home.

With your encouragement, new CNAs can learn to think the way the resident thinks—and it's worth it! It is possible to develop an almost automatic understanding of "difficult" behaviors. What's required is truly trying to put oneself in the cognitively impaired resident's place, and seeing the world as he or she sees it.

This understanding can lead to *action*. By making a thoughtful attempt to understand the meaning behind behavior, we can come up with new and more effective caring interventions.

Let's take the case of a resident who is sitting in the hallway, screaming continually. Both staff and other residents are becoming irritated, and the resident herself is clearly unhappy. How would a person-centered approach respond to this situation? Remember, this approach emphasizes understanding the meaning behind behaviors.

 WRITE on the board the ideas from the group.

 Now SAY:

These are all great ideas! Let's see how this can help a new CNA to provide better care.

First, keeping in mind that behaviors have meaning, staff can assess why this could be happening. Knowing the resident as much as possible, what activity would be *meaningful for the resident* and redirect the resident? Is the resident expressing a need for sensory stimulation? How can these needs be met? Gentle massage? Giving the resident a textured blanket or stuffed animal? Does she need to be toileted, or is she hungry or thirsty? Bored?

Is she in pain or discomfort? (What chronic illnesses does the resident suffer from that are likely associated with chronic pain?) By observing the resident and seeing how she responds to these kinds of interventions, the underlying need that stimulates the behavior can be identified. After several such times that the resident's behavior has been successfully interpreted—that is, the resident appears physically and emotionally comfortable—this "information" should be placed on the resident's plan of care so that her needs can be anticipated in the future.

This is what the person-centered approach adds to communication. The behaviors of residents, and especially persons with dementia, must be looked at in fresh, new ways. You will help the new CNA immensely if you help him or her look for the meaning behind resident behaviors and work with other staff to come up with creative solutions.

To conclude, SAY:

As a mentor, you will give valuable feedback to new CNAs on a regular basis. Your feedback is one of the primary means for the new CNA to know how he or she is doing. If new CNAs are not given clear feedback when it's necessary, they may develop some hard-to-break bad habits. Effective feedback gives the new CNA an anchor in a confusing sea of new responsibilities. It helps the CNA know what he or she is doing right and what areas need improvement.

Stress Management

Objectives of this Module

Mentors will:

- Learn to identify and practice effective ways to reduce stress
- Identify unsuccessful ways of dealing with stress
- Learn to help their mentees cope with stress
- Recognize and check themselves for signs of stress
- Learn to reduce stress by managing time more effectively

TOPIC #1

Managing Stress

 To begin, SAY:

As we have mentioned before, one of the primary goals of this mentoring program is to reduce staff turnover by giving new CNAs the resources they need to succeed. You were chosen as mentors because of the valuable resources you possess, resources that new CNAs can benefit from. These resources are not just made up of your caregiving and interpersonal skills. They also include the way you handle adversity, the way you bounce back from negative experiences and get back in the game—in short, the way you manage stress.

In surveys, over two-thirds of nursing assistants report high levels of stress on the job. As you well know, nursing homes are one of the most stressful working environments around. But stress doesn't have to lead to job frustration and burnout.

Part of your future success as a mentor will depend on your ability to help the new CNA develop strategies to stay motivated, manage stress, and find continuing job satisfaction. Being a nursing assistant is hard on the body, mind, emotions, and spirit. Acknowledging the difficulty of the job is one of the first steps to decreasing the stress of it. Some find it difficult to talk about stress, but talking about it is important. Talking about stress is healthy and keeps us from bottling it up inside.

As a mentor, you should offer new CNAs ideas for beating stress and recharging their batteries when the job gets them down. Being prepared for the inevitable stress of the job can help avoid the downward spiral of unhappiness and eventual burnout.

WRITE on the board:

- Is it possible to lower your job stress?

- What is your biggest source of job stress?

- What do you do to keep from carrying work stress home, and your home stress to work?

- What do you do to relax and enjoy yourself?

- Whom do you talk to at work when you're stressed?

Break the class into pairs. One person will be the interviewer and the other the interviewee. First, have the interviewee give answers to the questions on the board (listed above). Then, have the pairs reverse roles after a few minutes. After everyone has had time to answer, have a class discussion about the results. List everyone's answers on the board and see which are mentioned most. Write the top five answers on a list titled "Stress Reduction Tips."

A Hot Idea

For reducing stress:

Stress sometimes sneaks up on us gradually, and before we know it, we can end up feeling overwhelmed. One instant stress relief technique is to focus on breathing. Stress causes your breathing to become shallow, making you feel more stressed. To avoid this cycle, take time when you're feeling stressed to breathe deeply and restore your sense of calm. Try the following simple breathing exercise with your class:

1. Let's start by getting in a comfortable sitting position. Now put your hands in your lap and close your eyes.

2. Breathe in through your nose while you slowly count from one to five.

3. Release the breath at the same slow pace, counting backward from five to one.

4. Repeat this exercise a few times—In 1, 2, 3, 4, 5; Out 5, 4, 3, 2, 1.

5. Now, slowly open your eyes.

Ask the class members how they feel. Do people feel more relaxed, more at ease? Is this exercise something they can incorporate into their work-life occasionally?

To continue, SAY:

We've talked about some of your favorite stress reduction tips and learned this new one. Now, let's talk about how this relates to the new CNA.

Discussing stress can be an important part of your relationship with the new CNA. It will help you determine when "enough is enough" and show the CNA that you're interested in him or her as a person.

How will you know when your new CNA is under a lot of stress? Many people insist that they're okay when they're not. A few warning signs of stress are the following:

- Excessive emotions about unimportant things
- Constant irritability
- Disorganization
- Frequently arriving late

To find out where the stress is coming from, you should be supportive and nonthreatening to the new CNA. Many people don't want to discuss their personal problems, even if the problems are job-related. Some people think talking about stress is a sign of weakness. Emphasize that you respect the new CNA's privacy and that you are there to help him or her at work while he or she sorts out any personal issues.

It is impossible to live fully without experiencing stress. The following handout lists some stress techniques that don't work. These are stress traps that many people fall into. If you know what to look for, you can help a new CNA who seems to be falling into one of these traps.

 DISTRIBUTE Handout 5-1: Stress Traps.

 After reviewing the handout, SAY:

Let's look at an example of a new caregiver in trouble and see how we might be helpful.

DISTRIBUTE Handout 5-2: Gwen in Trouble.

Have a class discussion about Gwen's situation. Work together to answer the following questions:

- *As mentors, how would they help Gwen?*
- *Which aspects of their job as mentors would come into play in helping Gwen?*
- *How would they express concern about her work performance while also showing sensitivity to her home situation?*
- *What could they say to her?*
- *Should they get other help for Gwen (CNA supervisor, charge nurse, etc.)?*

 Then SAY:

Next, we're going to look at time management skills, another tool in fighting stress and burnout. Before we do that, though, let's try a little exercise that will demonstrate how to keep stress from overwhelming us. It can help you and the new CNAs that you will mentor. It's a way to check yourself for signs of stress. And awareness is one of the first steps in beating stress.

 DISTRIBUTE Handout 5-3: Take the BETS Check.

 To continue, SAY:

BETS stands for Body, Emotions, Thoughts, and Spirit—the four main parts of a person. BETS is a technique to help you see if you're under stress and understand where the stress lies, so you can begin to deal with it.

Give yourself the BETS Check whenever you feel that "something's wrong." It can help you find where the discomfort is coming from, so you can begin to solve the problem. Often, people misinterpret where the stress is coming from and don't get to the root of the real problem. You may think you're frustrated with your husband when you're really upset about an incident at work. You may want to ignore what the real problem is because it's too difficult or painful.

When we ignore a stressful problem, it can affect our physical well-being, showing up as a headache, backache, or stomachache. To avoid additional problems and discomfort, it's important to get to the real root of the problem. After using the BETS Check a few times yourself, plan to share it with the new CNA, as well as with your coworkers.

TOPIC #2

Managing Time

 To begin, SAY:

Sometimes, the problem is as simple as time, or the lack of it.

One of the best ways to cut down on stress is finding ways to manage your time. There's no question, good time management leads to less stress, which means less chance of job burnout. How can you practice good time management?

To manage time means to use it as efficiently as possible. The most important time management tool is learning how to prioritize. This means listing your tasks or activities from the most immediate and important to the least important.

In your work as a nursing assistant, your first priority must always be the immediate physical and emotional needs of your residents. Paying close attention to their care plans and individual needs is the best way to organize your schedule. You should also take into account your and your supervisor's goals and objectives.

Do you find that the new CNA seems under continuous strain, faced with one disaster after another? Does the new CNA seem unable to plan well to meet his or her learning and work goals? If you answer "yes" to either of these questions, then the new CNA probably needs help prioritizing.

Now, let's look at some proven tips for managing time well.

 DISTRIBUTE Handout 5-4: Time Management Tips.

 To conclude, SAY:

Remember, to teach the new CNA, you must do these things yourself. You must model them. If you're going to "talk the talk" with new CNAs, you also need to "walk the walk."

Stress can be contagious. A stressed-out role model can lead to a stressed-out new CNA. Don't just help the new CNA use the stress skills and time management tips in this module, use them yourself! Once you incorporate these stress-reducing techniques into your regular routine, they will become second nature to you and you will become a much calmer person!

MODULE 6

Your Job as a Mentor

Objectives of this Module

Mentors will:

- Understand the duties and responsibilities of a mentor
- Learn what is expected of them during the new CNA's critical "break-in" period and beyond
- Be able to administer the New CNA Evaluation form
- Learn about providing ongoing support to the mentee
- Feel well-prepared to begin the job of mentor

TOPIC #1

The Mentor's Responsibilities

 To begin, SAY:

In the last five sessions we have had together, we have dis-
cussed the different functions of a mentor. In this last session, we'll review some of those functions and discuss what
things you will need to focus on in the new CNA's first week,
or "break-in period," as well as during the weeks and months
following. First, let's look at your mentor job description.

Your chief function as a mentor is to help new CNAs learn
how to function safely and effectively in the facility and to
provide the highest quality of resident care possible. Another
of your main functions is to help the new CNA succeed—not
just in your facility but also in the long-term care field in general—giving encouragement and support when it's needed.

 **DISTRIBUTE Handout 6-1: The Mentor's Primary
Responsibilities.**

*Review the handout and allow time for any class discussion.
Tell the class that you will now discuss the needs of the new
CNA (the mentee).*

 To continue, SAY:

A lot of research has been done to find out what may seem
apparent to you: People don't stay at a job if they don't like
the people they're working with. If they feel they don't fit
in, they will go somewhere else where they feel more at
home. This fact especially applies to new CNAs.

A nursing assistant's work is hard enough without the added pressure of a negative social environment. If a new CNA feels unwelcome, that he or she has no one to talk to, or that no one cares about her or him, the new CNA will not usually stay. This is where the "act as social support for the new CNA" part of your job description comes into play.

 ASK the class the following questions and discuss the answers:

- Do you remember what it was like for you back when you were a new CNA?

- What kinds of social challenges did you face as a new CNA? How did you meet these challenges? Who helped you? What did they do that was helpful?

- Are there any "unwritten rules" on your unit that the new CNA should know about?

- Are there any CNAs on your unit who seem especially willing to help get the new CNA off to a good start?

- Are there others with whom the new CNA might carpool or travel with to work?

- Are there any ongoing communication problems on your unit that it might be help the new CNA to know about? How could you tactfully make the new CNA aware of these?

- What specific things can you think to do to make the new CNA feel welcome, instead of shut out?

- How can you encourage others on your unit to join in the welcoming process?

TOPIC #2

Week 1: The Break-in Period

 To begin, SAY:

"Put your best foot forward." This piece of wisdom applies to all beginnings—a new relationship, a new neighborhood, a new job. The first impression or early experience of someone can define a future. The first week of a new CNA's employment is extremely important for this reason. In this "break-in period"—which is the primary focus of this mentoring program—you can do a great deal to shape the new CNA's future success in the facility.

In this mentoring program there are two distinct periods of the mentoring relationship:

1. Week 1, known as the Break-in Period, and

2. Weeks 2 through 4, which we call the period of "Integration Into the Caregiving Team."

Let's start by looking closely at Week 1 and the crucial responsibilities and duties you will have. Remember, this is the time, this first week, when your role as mentor is critically important.

 DISTRIBUTE Handout 6-2: Mentor Responsibilities— Beginning of Week 1 and Handout 6-3: Mentor Responsibilities—Middle of Week 1.

 To continue, SAY:

Here's where "the rubber meets the road." These two handouts outline your primary responsibilities as mentors, so please take some time and look over each one carefully.

Next, read each handout aloud, one at a time, and review carefully. Spend whatever time is necessary reviewing the handouts and addressing any of the class's questions or concerns to ensure that everyone clearly understands what is expected of them.

DISTRIBUTE Handout 6-4: Mentor Responsibilities—End of Week 1.

Read aloud and review the handout carefully.

To continue, SAY:

These will be your responsibilities at the end of the first week. They are very important. First, let's look at the two evaluation forms.

DISTRIBUTE Handout 2-5: New CNA Evaluation and Handout 2-6: Mentor Evaluation.

Note: Handouts 2-5 and 2-6 are found in Module 2: Mentor as Teacher.

Review these two handouts. Remind the class that three different signatures are required because these two evaluations represent a communication between the mentor, the new CNA, and the mentors' supervisor. Remind mentors that the purpose of these evaluations is to guarantee the new CNA's success—and that they should fill in the evaluations in a truthful but encouraging, rather than critical, manner.

Then SAY:

Now, let's look at the last point in Handout 6-4, where it says "Most importantly . . ." It is here, at the end of the CNA's first week, where you, the mentor, and your supervisor must meet and decide how you and your new CNA will work together in the coming weeks. It is at this point where the two of you need to agree on how far your CNA has progressed as a caregiver, and what he or she will need from you in the next and final period of your mentoring relationship.

TOPIC #3

Weeks 2–4: Integration Into the Caregiving Team

 To begin, SAY:

The first week of the mentoring relationship is the most important and is the time that the most is expected of the mentor. But this brief period of intense help and support is, in most cases, not enough for the new CNA.

Ongoing support—over the course of Weeks 2, 3, and 4, and perhaps beyond—is necessary to help the new CNA become an excellent caregiver and fully integrated into the caregiving team. The question at this point is: How much and what kind of support?

The evaluation that the mentor and the mentor's supervisor make regarding the new CNA's progress at the end of Week 1 will determine the nature of this support for the next three weeks, this time we call the period of "integration into the caregiving team." Depending on the evaluation and how much the mentor and the CNA will need to interact, here is a list of the possible responsibilities of the mentor.

DISTRIBUTE Handout 6-5: Possible Mentor Responsibilities—Weeks 2–4.

 To continue, SAY:

You notice how the handout reads "possible" mentor responsibilities? That's because, at the end of Week 1, you and your supervisor will determine what your specific responsibilities will be over the next three weeks to help ensure that your new CNA gains independence and becomes an excellent caregiver. You two will decide how much, and in what way, you and your CNA will interact during this second and final phase.

As a minimum, you will meet regularly with your CNA, at least once a week, so that he or she continues to receive your help and support.

Review the handout and discuss how this second phase will vary depending on what the mentor's new CNA still needs.

 DISTRIBUTE Handout 6-6: Mentor Responsibilities— End of Month 1.

Read the handout aloud.

 To continue, SAY:

This moment—at the end of the first month—marks the conclusion of the formal mentoring arrangement. If you, your supervisor, and the new CNA all feel that the new CNA has gained full independence and is ready to "go out on his or her own," then stop, take a moment, and congratulate your CNA for coming a long way!

Make sure you explain to your class that this doesn't mean that they have to stop seeing or meeting with their CNA. In fact, if it is possible within your facility, you should encourage them to continue to see and support their mentees whenever possible.

Also explain that if the mentor's supervisor or the mentor feel that the formal mentor relationship needs to continue in some capacity, then it should, if at all possible. If the new CNA stills needs ongoing support and help from the mentor, then arrangements should be made.

Please note: Make sure that every one of your mentors has copies of all the handouts in this module, and intends to hold onto and refer to them as they begin their duties as mentors.

Congratulations! You and your class have now completed the mentoring program!

End this module with some form of celebration to mark your accomplishment. You may use any, or all, of the suggestions below to recognize those who have participated. You may have additional ideas of your own.

- *Have a graduation ceremony or celebration where participants are officially declared "Mentors" or "CNA Mentors." You may want to include your facility's name in the title.*

- *Have your administrator hand out certificates to the new mentors.*

- *Give each graduate a pin or patch to wear saying "Mentor" or "CNA Mentor." You may want to include your facility's name.*

- *Have your administrator and/or DON prepare some remarks about the program, the facility, and the role of the new mentors.*

- *Take pictures of each new mentor, as well as the entire group; post in a prominent location in the facility.*

- *In closing remarks, tell the mentors that the facility is counting on them to shape new generations of CNAs.*

- *Emphasize that their supervisors will be working closely with them and be available to address questions, concerns, or problems.*

- *Express your gratitude for their commitment to the facility and their careers, and confidence in their abilities.*

- *Tell the class that there will be a follow-up "booster session" after several weeks, in which they will be able to discuss their experiences. Ideally, the booster session should take place during the third week of the mentoring program.*

MODULE 7

A Booster Session for Mentors

Objectives of this Module

Mentors will:

- Review key points from the earlier sessions of this program

- Identify problems and successes that have come up in their mentoring experience

- Brainstorm ideas for improving the mentoring program

Introduction

For The Instructor Only

Research has shown that training programs like this one can benefit from what is called a "booster session." The idea behind this session is to meet with all mentors in a group session that allows them to discuss any difficulties that have come up in the mentoring process, as well as successes they have experienced. It is also useful to review some of the main points of the previous sessions, to reinforce basic principles of the mentoring program.

In this session, you will provide the mentors with several handouts from previous sessions, review them, and discuss them. In particular, you will review the activities the mentors were to accomplish (from Module 6). It is important for you to understand whether the mentors were able to complete the activities, and if not, what difficulties were encountered. In the group setting, more successful mentors can help "mentor" others who are encountering challenges.

Make this booster session positive, relaxed, and enjoyable. Provide lunch or refreshments and create a celebratory atmosphere: By this time, your mentors will be well along in the process and are likely to have positive accomplishments to report. It is important as well to allow the mentors to openly express any frustration or difficulties they may have experienced. If a mentor reports serious or ongoing problems in the mentoring relationship, be sure to work one-on-one with him or her later to resolve issues that cannot be fully addressed in the booster session.

We suggest that the booster session be conducted when two weeks of mentoring training has been completed, or as close to the mid-point of the mentoring relationships as possible.

TOPIC #1

Review of Key Points about Mentoring

 To begin, SAY:

Our session today is different from the other ones we had before you began mentoring. Our goal today is to do a quick refresher of some of the important concepts and ideas in earlier training sessions. Then we're going to take a look at your mentoring experience so far and check in on any challenges that may have come up in working with your mentees.

Now I'm going to do a quick review of some key points about mentoring.

In the remainder of this part of the booster session, distribute and briefly review the following handouts. Hand them out in the order indicated, and quickly note the content of the earlier training module that relates to the handout. You will need to review the previous sessions in the manual in preparation for this presentation.

Note: From your discussions with the mentors, you may have learned that another topic should be reviewed. If so, you may substitute another topic for the ones suggested here. This review should take about 10 minutes.

Handout 1-1: Definition of a Mentor

Handout 1-3: The Three Functions of a Mentor

Handout 4-3: Guidelines for Active Listening

Handout 4-4: Tips for Good Feedback

Handout 6-1: The Mentor's Primary Responsibilities

You do not need to specifically ask group members about each of these slides. The goal is to help focus the discussion by reminding them of key skills and responsibilities. However, you should ask if they have any comments when you have finished.

TOPIC #2

Review of the Mentoring Experience

 To begin, SAY:

Now, I would like learn more about the kinds of things you did during these first few weeks as a mentor. Let's look at the handouts about mentor responsibilities; you will remember that we went over these in the last session of your mentor training program.

Of course, any list like this is an ideal, and the reality of being a mentor will be different from that ideal. I'm sure there are some activities that you and your mentor did together, and others that did not work out. In addition, I bet that some of the activities went well, and others may not have worked or were disappointing. Our goal today is to learn from one another about what worked well and what might need some improvement.

 DISTRIBUTE Handout 6-2: Mentor Responsibilities— Beginning of Week 1.

 Now SAY:

Let's look at these four activities. Were you able to do these activities? How did they go? Which ones worked well and which ones didn't?

Be sure to allow all CNAs to respond. If someone does not speak up, you can ask (without insisting) what his or her experience was like.

Now SAY:

That's great feedback! Now let's look at the rest of the mentoring activities. Did these take place like the handout suggests? Any problems come up for you?

REPEAT FOR Handout 6-3: Mentor Responsibilities—Middle of Week 1.

REPEAT FOR Handout 6-4: Mentor Responsibilities—End of Week 1.

REPEAT FOR Handout 6-5: Possible Mentor Responsibilities—Weeks 2–4.

REPEAT FOR Handout 6-6: Mentor Responsibilities—End of Month 1.

Note: The handouts you review will depend on when you are holding this booster session. For example, if two weeks have gone by, you will not review Handout 6-6.

 WRITE on the board the main issues or problems that came up.

Ask the group members for ways they handled the problem or issue that is raised. Be sure in the group setting to maintain an open and nonjudgmental attitude. If you are concerned about an individual mentor's approach, you can mention this to the group in a nonthreatening way, and follow up with the individual mentor after the session.

If individuals did not complete a component of the program that you believe is important, engage the rest of the group for suggestions for these individuals. Use the group session as joint problem-solving for issues mentors are having.

TOPIC #3

Visioning Exercise

 SAY:

I'd like to conclude this session by getting your ideas for how to make the program better.

 DISTRIBUTE: Sheets of paper or note cards.

 SAY:

I'd like you to write down as many answers to the following question as you like. I'm not going to ask you to hand these in; this is just for you to put down your first thoughts on the question. It will help us discuss your ideas.

Here's the question: **Based on your experience so far as a mentor, what can we do to improve the Mentoring Program?**

Please write down whatever you think, and don't worry whether it seems feasible or not. Our goal here is just to brainstorm ideas that might make the program better.

WAIT 2–3 minutes while group members write down answers.

 SAY:

Okay, let's begin: Who has an idea for improving or changing the program?

WRITE all ideas on the board.

Discuss the ideas that have been suggested. When all suggestions have been listed, ask these questions:

- Which of these ideas seem most important to you? Which seem less important?

- Are there any of these ideas we can start right away?

 To conclude, SAY:

Thank you so much for your feedback on the program. I'm going to take all of your suggestions and we will consider them very carefully. Please remember that I am available to discuss any issues you are having in your role as mentors. The work you are doing as mentors is extremely important for our facility, and we are all very grateful!

CNA
MENTORING
MADE
EASY

Program Curriculum Handouts

HANDOUT 1-1

Definition of Mentor

MENTOR:

A person who takes a special interest in helping someone else learn, develop, and succeed.

HANDOUT 1-2

Overview of the Mentor's Job

As a mentor, your responsibilities will include many, if not all, of the following:

⮑ **1. Welcoming the new CNA**
- Introducing yourself and other staff members
- Inviting the new CNA into social groups. (e.g., lunch, after work, etc.)
- Directing the new CNA's learning experience
- Listening to the new CNA and showing interest in the CNA as a person
- Being an advocate for the new CNA
- Helping solve problems

⮑ **2. Providing continuous constructive feedback**
- Reinforcing the positive, discussing the negative
- Focusing on behavior rather than on the person
- Describing rather than judging
- Involving your supervisor at the first sign of a problem
- Providing support

⮑ **3. Being a model of clinical competence**
- Possessing excellent clinical skills
- Following facility policies, procedures, and the proper use of facility resources
- Presenting a positive image for a CNA

HANDOUT 1-2 *continued*

Overview of the Mentor's Job *continued*

↶ **4. Teaching clinical skills**
- Assessing the new CNA's needs
- Formulating goals with the new CNA
- Evaluating your teaching skills and seeking assistance for improvement
- Daily planning with the new CNA and working with him or her to achieve it

↶ **5. Documenting the new CNA's ability to perform skills and procedures**
- Talking with the new CNA and your supervisor to assess the CNA's progress
- Using established evaluation forms to document progress

↶ **6. Providing information and clinical guidance**
- Making sure the new CNA knows where you are or what plans you have made for him or her, if you are not available
- Explaining unit routines
- Making realistic demands based on the person's progress, and increasing expectations as the person progresses
- Working with the new CNA to provide all the information necessary to carry out assignments
- Always answering and encouraging questions

HANDOUT 1-3

The Three Functions of a Mentor

⊃   1. Teacher

⊃   2. Role model

⊃   3. Supporter

HANDOUT 2-1

Definition of Learning

LEARNING:

To acquire knowledge of a
subject or skill as a result
of study, experience, or
instruction.

HANDOUT 2-2

The Four Types of Learners

1. The VISUAL Learner
- Learns by seeing things being done
- Likes to watch demonstrations
- Prefers face-to-face meetings
- Thinks in pictures
- Reads emotions by facial expressions

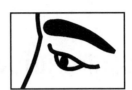

2. The AUDITORY Learner
- Learns by hearing instructions
- Likes things clearly explained to them in words
- Likes music and talking on the telephone
- Talks about situations and possibilities
- Enjoys hearing self and others talk

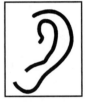

3. The THINKING Learner
- Learns by working things out in her head
- Likes written directions that she can study
- Likes to put things in categories
- Enjoys problem solving
- Learns by asking questions

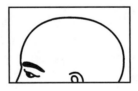

4. The HANDS-ON Learner
- Learns by trial and error
- Likes to try things on her own until she gets it right
- Uses gestures when speaking
- Enjoys performing various physical activities
- Expresses emotions by using body language

HANDOUT 2-3

Definition of Teaching

TEACHING:

To show someone the way;
to direct or guide.

To communicate knowledge.

HANDOUT 2-4

Definition of Evaluate

EVALUATE:

To ascertain or fix the value or worth of something.

To examine or judge carefully.

HANDOUT 2-5

New CNA Evaluation

☞ **New CNA Evaluation—to be filled out by Mentor.**

Name of New CNA: _____ Unit: _____ Date:

Name of Mentor: _____Title: _____

For End of Week 1 _____	For End of Month 1 ____

Rate the new CNA in each category:

1—Excellent
2—Good
3—Acceptable
4—Needs Improvement
5—Requires Immediate Attention
NA—Not Applicable

WORK QUALITY
- Completes assignments in allotted time _____
- Provides quality care _____
- Assists other staff _____
- Works safely at all times _____
- Follows infection control procedures _____
- Communicates effectively with residents, staff, families _____
- Respects residents rights _____

JOB PROFICIENCY
- Understands duties and responsibilities _____
- Organizes and plans work _____
- Performs skills correctly _____
- Knowledge of care plans _____

DEPENDABILITY
- Is prompt and has good attendance _____
- Notifies staff when leaving/returning to unit _____
- Returns from breaks and meals on time _____

ATTITUDE
- Shows motivation and ambition _____
- Eager to learn _____
- Accepts direction and training _____
- Shows respect for residents, staff, families _____

TO LIST SPECIFIC RECOMMENDATIONS OR ADDITIONAL COMMENTS, USE BACK OF FORM ➡

_____   _____
Mentor Signature   **Date**

_____   _____
New CNA (mentee) Signature   **Date**

_____   _____
Mentor's Supervisor Signature   **Date**

HANDOUT 2-6

Mentor Evaluation

☞ **Mentor Evaluation—<u>to be filled out by new CNA.</u>**

Name of Mentor: _____ Title: _____ Date: _____

Name of New CNA: _____ Unit: _____

| For End of Week 1 _____ | For End of Month 1 ____ |

	YES	NO
• My Mentor made me feel welcome and introduced me to other staff.	___	___
• My Mentor encouraged me to ask questions and was available to answer them.	___	___
• My Mentor explained new procedures and equipment to me.	___	___
• My Mentor gave me praise for what I did correctly.	___	___
• My Mentor encouraged me in learning my role on the unit.	___	___

TO LIST SPECIFIC RECOMMENDATIONS OR ADDITIONAL COMMENTS, USE BACK OF FORM ➜

_____   Date
New CNA (mentee) Signature

_____   Date
Mentor Signature

_____   Date
Mentor's Supervisor Signature

HANDOUT 3-1

A Leader Is . . .

⊃ A Decision-maker

⊃ A Problem-solver

⊃ An Organizer

⊃ A Priority-setter

HANDOUT 3-2

Definition of a Role Model

ROLE MODEL:

Person who is looked to by others as an example to be imitated.

HANDOUT 3-3

Two Primary Leadership Styles

FACILITATIVE LEADERS:

- Interact often with followers
- Ask questions to solve problems
- Collaborate with followers to find joint solutions
- Work well in team settings
- Practice good listening
- Demonstrate patience and willingness to help others
- Provide frequent follow-ups
- Negotiate assignments

DIRECTIVE LEADERS:

- Do not emphasize personal interactions
- Provide answers to problems
- Like to talk more than listen
- Closely monitor followers
- Make plans and decisions alone
- Give detailed instructions
- Place emphasis on rules and regulations
- Feel comfortable in hierarchical settings

HANDOUT 3-4

Leadership Style: Scenario 1

SCENARIO #1

Louis is a new CNA who has recently transferred from the kitchen staff. He is doing a satisfactory job and trying very hard. He is very dependable and seems eager to succeed in his new position. As you walk down the hall of the unit one evening, you notice him yelling at a resident with Alzheimer's who doesn't want to take her bath. You remember that over the past few days, you've seen him yell at other residents and get easily frustrated at least two different times. As Louis's mentor, which leadership traits (listed in Handout 3-3) would be most effective for addressing this situation, and why?

_____

_____

_____

_____

_____

_____

HANDOUT 3-5

Leadership Style: Scenario #2

SCENARIO #2

Sarah, a new CNA, is well liked by her coworkers and residents. She is cheerful, upbeat, and a good communicator, but she has a serious problem with her organizing skills. You notice that she is sometimes forgetful about filling out necessary paperwork. Although she was warned about her poorly managed time and lateness two days ago, no improvement can be seen. The holidays are coming up and you are worried about whether or not she can be depended on to show up for her shift. As Sarah's mentor, which leadership traits (listed in Handout 3-3) would be most effective for addressing this situation, and why?

_____

_____

_____

_____

_____

_____

HANDOUT 3-6

Leadership Style: Scenario #3

SCENARIO #3

Cathy, a new caregiver who has been at the facility for a little over a month, proves to be a good learner and conscientious caregiver. She has just received a good one-month evaluation, but her coworkers still don't seem to like her. They have started to gossip about her behind her back and make fun of her superior attitude, because she often makes suggestions and does her work extremely carefully. Yesterday, you observed her telling Julia, an older CNA who has been working in the facility for 20 years, how to lift a resident. As Cathy's mentor, which leadership traits (listed in Handout 3-3) would be most effective for addressing this situation, and why?

_____

_____

_____

_____

_____

_____

HANDOUT 3-7

Leadership Style: Scenario #4

SCENARIO #4

Mia is a new CNA who is quiet and hard to get to know. You aren't sure whether she likes her new job or not. There is a fire alarm in the dining room while you and Mia are assisting a resident with eating difficulties. Many of the other CNAs ignore it, assume it's only a fire drill, and don't interrupt their activities to leave the building. Mia watches them, follows their lead, and continues to help the resident eat. As Mia's mentor, which leadership traits (listed in Handout 3-3) would be most effective for addressing this situation, and why?

_____

_____

_____

_____

_____

_____

HANDOUT 4-1

The Elements of Communication

There are three elements in
every communication:

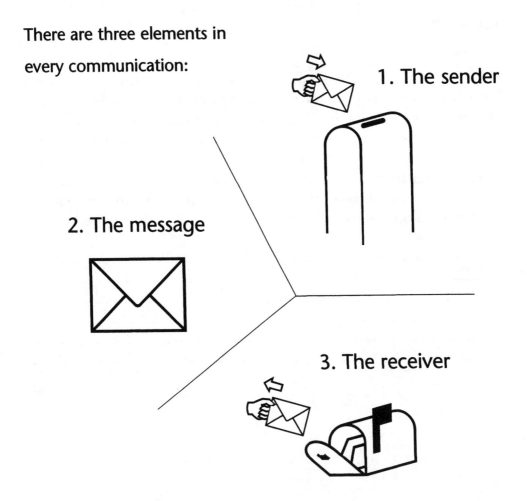

1. The sender

2. The message

3. The receiver

HANDOUT 4-2

Definition of Active Listening

ACTIVE LISTENING:

Understanding what the sender of a message is thinking and feeling.

HANDOUT 4-3

Guidelines for Active Listening

1. INITIATE

- Make the speaker feel welcome and respected
- Offer "door openers," opportunities to talk

2. CLARIFY

- Ask questions to make sure you understand speaker's message
- Repeat back the message in your own words

3. SUPPORT

- Look for the feelings behind the message
- Have relaxed, attentive posture and comfortable eye contact
- Show your human side. Let the speaker know if you have faced the same problem

4. FOLLOW-UP

- Offer other resources to help with the problem
- Help the speaker identify the possible next step

HANDOUT 4-4

Tips for Good Feedback

⊃ Focus on the behavior, not the person

⊃ Be specific rather than general

⊃ Be supportive

⊃ Emphasize what's possible and beneficial

⊃ Take timing into account

⊃ Invite feedback on the feedback

HANDOUT 5-1

Stress Traps

1. USING UNHEALTHY STRESS STRATEGIES

People often worsen their stress by using strategies such as smoking, drinking, and overeating, which actually make things worse. These strategies might offer quick relief but hurt more in the long run.

2. BEING A PERFECTIONIST

Setting expectations for themselves that are too high can overwhelm CNAs. As a mentor, you can help by putting the job into perspective. Remind them that they should do the best possible job without threatening their physical or emotional health.

3. ISOLATING YOURSELF

Many CNAs are caregivers both at work and at home and can sometimes feel isolated in their ongoing struggles. Reassure them by reminding them that they are not alone. Help them to find solutions and listen to their problems.

HANDOUT 5-2

Gwen in Trouble

Gwen, a new CNA, has been at the facility for three weeks and received a very good one-week evaluation. She is a warm person who has a lot of enthusiasm for her new job and enjoys being with the residents. She started out as an energetic and dependable worker, but lately things have started to change due to family problems.

Gwen's decision to become a nursing assistant was a difficult one. Her husband is a man of old-fashioned values, who doesn't believe that women should work. Because the family was struggling to get by on just his salary and their son was about to graduate from high school, Gwen decided that she should earn extra money.

Their son, upset by his parents' fighting, has started getting into trouble at school, mouthing off to teachers and fighting with students. Last week, he hit another boy and was suspended from school. Afraid that his problems will increase, Gwen fears that she may have to quit her job.

Her husband has been pressuring her to quit and she has grown more and more upset. Her work has been suffering. She has been forgetful in her duties and is becoming distant with her coworkers and the residents. Yesterday she started crying because the nurse manager reminded her to answer a call light that had been flashing for some time.

Gwen is so overwhelmed, she doesn't know what to do or where to turn. Her roles as wife, mother, and CNA are all in question.

As her mentor, how could you help Gwen?

HANDOUT 5-3

Take the BETS Check

Take a minute to check yourself for signs of stress. Sit somewhere comfortable, take a deep breath, and ask yourself the following questions:

⊃ **BODY**
- Have I had enough sleep?
- Do I need to exercise?
- Am I hungry or did I overeat?
- Did I drink too much coffee or sodas?
- What can I do to make my body more comfortable?

⊃ **EMOTIONS**
- What am I feeling right now?
- Are these feelings familiar?
- Can I name these different feelings?
- Do my feelings come from my current situation, or are they left over from a past one?

⊃ **THOUGHTS**
- What thoughts are running through my head?
- Am I speaking disrespectfully to myself, judging myself harshly?
- Am I "awfulizing," or exaggerating how bad things are?
- Am I assuming the worst or imagining a bleak future?

⊃ **SPIRIT**
- Have I forgotten what's most important to me?
- Do I need to remind myself of my purpose? Of my worth?
- What is most meaningful to me?

HANDOUT 5-4

Time Management Tips

TIME MANAGEMENT TIPS FOR THE NEW CNA

⊃ Arrive a few minutes before your shift.

⊃ Make a list of things that need to be accomplished and cross them off when you finish them.

⊃ Number the list with highest priorities at the top.

⊃ Consolidate tasks when possible.

⊃ Allow time for accurate documentation.

⊃ Do what's necessary when you think of it, or write it down so you'll remember it later.

⊃ Be flexible and remember: Interruptions and crises are part of the job.

HANDOUT 6-1

The Mentor's Primary Responsibilities

THE MENTOR'S PRIMARY RESPONSIBILITIES INCLUDE:

- Help in the new CNA's orientation
- Act as social support for the new CNA
- Contribute to a positive learning environment for new CNAs
- Identify and meet the new CNA's learning needs
- Gradually increase the resident care assignments for the new CNA, as appropriate
- Offer your clinical knowledge to the new CNA
- Make sure the new CNA follows facility policies and procedures
- Fill out all evaluation forms and other facility documentation, as necessary
- Help the new CNA gain gradual independence
- Be a leader in the facility
- Be an available resource for at least one month to the new CNA, and longer if possible
- Modify and adapt the program, with other mentors, to meet your facility's needs

HANDOUT 6-2

Mentor Responsibilities—Beginning of Week 1

On the new CNA's first day, the mentor should:

➲ Give a comprehensive tour of the facility, especially of the unit.

➲ Introduce the new CNA to everyone on the unit, staff and residents.

➲ Explain breaks, meal assignments, and other basic employee policies.

➲ Address any initial concerns or problems the new CNA might have.

HANDOUT 6-3

Mentor Responsibilities—Middle of Week 1

During the new CNA's first week, the mentor should:

⊃ Have the new CNA "shadow" the mentor the first few days

⊃ Provide and supervise hands-on learning opportunities

⊃ Begin to give caregiving assignments to the new CNA

⊃ Accompany the new CNA to all meals and breaks

⊃ Offer feedback on a daily basis

⊃ Demonstrate any new procedures

⊃ Continue to increase the caregiving assignments, as appropriate

HANDOUT 6-4

Mentor Responsibilities—End of Week 1

At the end of the new CNA's first week, the mentor should:

⊃ Have the new CNA assigned to as much resident care as the mentor thinks the new CNA can comfortably handle

⊃ Fill out the New CNA Evaluation form (Handout 2-5)

⊃ Make sure the new CNA fills out the Mentor Evaluation form (Handout 2-6)

⊃ Meet with the mentors' supervisor and the new CNA to review and sign both evaluation forms. Most importantly, this is the time to reach an agreement on the new CNA's progress. Where does the new CNA still need help and support? How closely should the mentor and new CNA work together over the next three weeks? Have you clearly defined those areas where the new CNA still needs assistance?

HANDOUT 6-5

Possible Mentor Responsibilities—Weeks 2–4

WHAT DOES THE NEW CNA STILL NEED?

During this second and final mentoring phase—depending on what the new CNA needs—the mentor may do some, or all, of the following:

- Meet with the new CNA on a regular, scheduled basis to offer support, feedback, and to address any concerns or problems

- Provide and supervise hands-on learning opportunities

- Offer additional caregiving and clinical expertise

- Act as ongoing social support

- Intercede with others on the new CNA's behalf, if necessary

- Continue to increase the caregiving assignments, as appropriate, until the new CNA has a full resident care load

HANDOUT 6-6

Mentor Responsibilities—End of Month 1

At the end of the new CNA's first month, the mentor should:

⊃ Have the new CNA assigned to a full resident care load

⊃ Fill out the New CNA Evaluation form (Handout 2-5)

⊃ Make sure the new CNA fills out the Mentor Evaluation form (Handout 2-6)

⊃ Meet with the mentor's supervisor and the new CNA to review and sign both evaluation forms

Congratulate the new CNA!
(This marks the end of the formal mentoring arrangement, unless additional help is needed.)

CNA
MENTORING
MADE
EASY

Appendix 1:

Program Forms

Mentor Application Form

TO BE FILLED OUT BY THE EMPLOYEE

Name:_____ Job title: _____

What are the reasons why you would like to participate in the Mentoring Program? What do you think qualifies you to become a Mentor?

_____

_____

_____

_____

_____

_____

_____

_____

_____

_____

_____

I understand the rules established for the Mentoring Program for nursing assistants. I also understand that my absence from any training session associated with this program may constitute voluntary withdrawal from this program.

Employee's signature:_____ Date: _____

TO BE FILLED OUT BY THE FACILITY ADMINISTRATION

Employee's date of hire: _____ Employee's job title: _____

Does this employee meet our facility's eligibility
requirements for this program?   YES   NO

I recommend this employee for participation in the Mentoring Program:

Employee's supervisor: _____ Date: _____

Director of Nursing: _____ Date: _____

Graduation Certificate—*Sample Only*

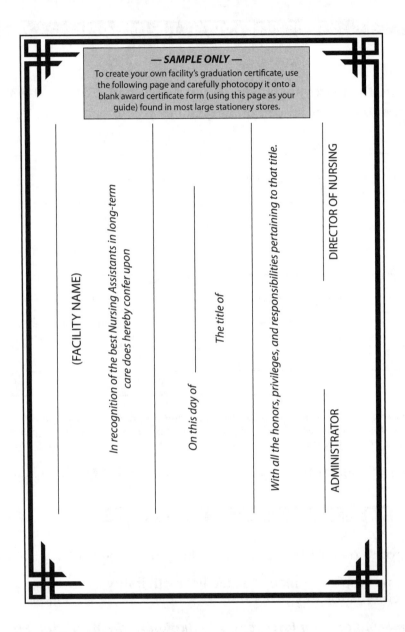

— SAMPLE ONLY —

To create your own facility's graduation certificate, use the following page and carefully photocopy it onto a blank award certificate form (using this page as your guide) found in most large stationery stores.

(FACILITY NAME)

In recognition of the best Nursing Assistants in long-term care does hereby confer upon

On this day of

The title of

With all the honors, privileges, and responsibilities pertaining to that title.

DIRECTOR OF NURSING

ADMINISTRATOR

Graduation Certificate—*Master*

(FACILITY NAME)

In recognition of the best Nursing Assistants in long-term care does hereby confer upon

On this day of

The title of

With all the honors, privileges, and responsibilities pertaining to that title.

DIRECTOR OF NURSING

ADMINISTRATOR